Sex, Chocolate & Alcohol Can Be Good For You

Professor Norman Ratcliffe

A catalogue record for this book is available from the British Library

ISBN: 978-1-907962-69-1

Published by Cranmore Publications

www.cranmorepublications.co.uk

Almost every day articles are being published on the evils of sex, chocolate and alcohol with possible health and social benefits of these pleasures poorly publicised.

This little book presents data that indicates that, in moderation, these activities may actually be beneficial. It is therefore recommended for people of most ages in the hope that it will be informative and help to provide a more balanced view of pleasures that are an integral part of most people's lives.

The Author

Professor Norman Ratcliffe is a founder member of a team that recently discovered a new antibiotic potentially capable of curing MRSA and *Clostridium difficile*. This work was presented to Prince Phillip at St. James's Palace, London and was the subject of major media attention in the UK on ITV News and in many leading newspapers, including the Wall Street Journal, around the World. He is a Fellow of the Royal Society of Medicine and has previously run a "Health Alert" blood-testing company. He has published over 200 books and research papers on immunology, cancer invasion, influenza, tropical diseases and MRSA. He played squash for Wales, ran the London Marathon at the age of 50 and works-out regularly in the gym.

Professor Ratcliffe retired recently after 25 years as a University Research Professor. He decided to finally complete his comprehensive book on health *"It's Your Life: End the Confusion From Inconsistent Health Advice"* after 5 years work in order to help the many people who are confused about health and fitness issues and who have constantly been asking his advice.

Contents

Contents

Introduction

We have all heard warnings before about sex, chocolate and alcohol such as:

"Too much sex can be dangerous for the heart and result in nasty infections"

or

"Eating chocolate rots the teeth and makes you fat"

or

"Alcohol is addictive, causes bad behaviour, destroys the liver and breaks up marriages"

Unfortunately, much of this bad press is associated with the bad behaviour of "famous" people with high profiles in television, politics or even the church.

Average people struggling to survive on minimal wages see the media headlines about their icons and may be tempted to copy these idols. This has led to going out and getting "plastered" seemingly being normalised.

This book attempts to present a more balanced view of sex, chocolate and alcohol and gives information about both the benefits and evils of these pleasures so that people can form their own opinions away from the media hype.

Chapter 1

Sex can be good for you

But only if precautions are taken to avoid the risks of unwanted pregnancies or infection.

We have all heard warnings before about sex such as:

"Too much sex can be dangerous for the heart and result in nasty infections"

Evidence indicates that, in moderation, sex can have many health benefits.

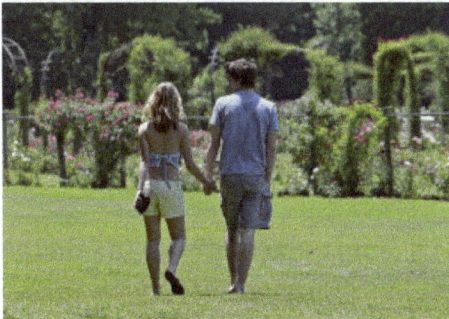

The benefits of sex have been reported to include:

1. Longer life-span

2. Reduced heart attacks
   (fewer cardiovascular problems)

3. Stress relief

4. Reduced depression

5. Improved bonding between people

6. Better sleep

7. Enhanced resistance to illness

8. Reduced risk of prostate and breast cancers

9. Burning calories and weight control

10. Miscellaneous benefits

Sex almost seems to be a cure-all medicine!

Unfortunately, little evidence of these benefits of sex is usually given in most reports. These reports are mainly published to capture headlines and sell newspapers and magazines. Irwin Goldstein, the editor of "Journal of Sexual Medicine" and an urologist, has been reported to have said that "more research is needed to evaluate all these claims" but such studies cost money and this is difficult to get for research on sex (quoted in The Wall Street Journal, ref 1). However, anyone who has been in a loving relationship can confirm the benefits of sex in terms of bonding and feelings of well-being without the need for confirmation from scientific evidence!

Longer life-span and reduced heart attacks

Sex increases the heart beat about the same amount as walking up two flights of stairs. Sex is therefore a beneficial exercise but insufficient to maintain fitness and health unless you are an insatiable sexual athlete! In addition, even if you have heart disease, the risk of a heart attack during sex is usually quite low as the exercise involved is usually only mild or moderate **unless you are being unfaithful and in an exotic or erotic environment (!)**. In addition, there is evidence that sexually active and faithful men have fewer cardiovascular problems and live longer. Also, the more frequent the sex (2-3 times per week compared with just once per month), the less the risk of heart attacks (2).

Stress relief and reduced depression

Additional benefits of "sex" include reductions in blood pressure, heart rate and stress simply by hugging or stroking your partner, although penetrative sex seems to be a greater de-stressor (3). People who have penile-vaginal intercourse have been shown to react less to stressful situations, such as public speaking and verbal arithmetic, than those who masturbate or have sex without penetration. Thus, having sexual intercourse just before an important speech may be beneficial!

In addition, in a preliminary study of female college students, it has been shown that those who had sex without the use of condoms had fewer symptoms of depression than those who used condoms regularly. Since it is known that semen contains a cocktail of hormones, such as testosterone, oestrogen and prostaglandins, it has been suggested that absorption of these by the wall of the vagina may not only control symptoms of depression but also promote further sexual activity (4). *I recommend reading*

"An ode to the many evolved virtues of human semen" by Jesse Berring (5) for more details.

Improved bonding between people

During sex, levels of hormones rapidly change and alter the behaviour of the participants. For example, dopamine increases result in arousal, desire and pair bonding. Dopamine activity is also elevated by other hormones, incuding oxytocin and vasopressin, which particularly affect pair bonding and monogamy. After orgasm, another hormone, prolactin, is also released, and with oxytocin and vasopressin, result in drowsiness to reduce sexual arousal (6). Thus, sex increases bonding and sleepiness.

Enhanced immunity and avoidance of illness and cancer

There is limited evidence that sex actually stimulates immunity. Thus, people who have sex 1-2 times (but not more than twice) per week have higher antibody levels than those who have no sex at all. This antibody is present in the nose and respiratory system and protects against colds, flu and other infectious agents in the air (7).

Sex, however, may protect the body against infectious agents and cancers, such as prostate and breast cancer, as it is a great de-stressor. Many studies show that stress and depression may impair the immune response and assist the spread of some types of viral infections (8) and cancer (9).

Finally, it has been shown that frequent ejaculation by 20-50 yr old men may reduce the risk of prostate cancer in later life by preventing the accumulation of carcinogens in the prostate gland (10). The results relied upon the men recalling orgasmic events many years previously so that the accuracy of the data is questionable. Similarly, men who ejaculated 21 or more times per month have lower prostate cancer risks in comparison with those with just 4-7 ejaculations monthly.

Burning calories and weight control

Since sex is usually regarded as only a mild or moderate exercise, the Calories burnt are about 133, 189 and 224, respectively, for people weighing 60, 86 and 102 kilos (11). Males apparently burn more calories than females but these figures are very general and certainly do not apply to the more enthusiastic people! However, sex does not usually figure as a reliable way of losing weight or staying fit.

Miscellaneous benefits

There are other miscellaneous benefits ascribed to sex with most requiring additional confirmation. Sex may thus relieve pain due to the production of oxytocin and endorphins after sex, enhance self-esteem, increase the sense of smell, reduce the risk of diabetes, slow the aging process, and strengthen the pelvic muscles to reduce the risk of incontinence.

Risks of sex

The benefits far outweigh the risks of safe sex. The main risk is that **unprotected sex** results in about 340 million cases of sexually transmitted diseases annually. Over 50% of these diseases occur in 15-24 yr olds and include chlamydia, hepatitis B, syphilis and AIDS with gonorrhoea also re-emerging. Another risk with unprotected sex is unplanned pregnancies with about 86 million in 2008. Finally, casual sexual encounters also result in countless divorces with untold stress and heartache.

Reference sources

1.http://online.wsj.com/.../SB1000142405274870 45694045762989533651206 30.html

2. Hall and colleagues, American Journal of Cardiology, Vol. 105, pages 192-197, 2010.

3. Brody, Biological Psychology, Vol. 71, pages 214-222, 2006.

4. Gallup and colleagues, Archives of Sexual Behaviour, Vol. 31, pages 289-293, 2002.

5.Berring, Scientific American blog, September 22nd, 2010.

6. Kruger and colleagues, Journal of Endocrinology, Vol. 179, pages357–365, 2003.

7. Charnetski and colleagues, Psychology Report, Vol. 94, pages 839-44, 2004.

8. Kemeny and Schedlowski, Brain, Behaviour and Immunity, Vol. 21, pages 1009-1018, 2007.

9. Reiche and colleagues, Lancet Oncocology, Vol. 5, pages 617-25, 2004.

10. Giles and colleagues, British Journal of Urology International, Vol. 92, pages 211-216, 2003.

11. Ratcliffe, <u>It's Your Life, End the Confusion from Inconsistent Health Advice</u>, Cranmore Publications, 2011.

Chapter 2

Chocolate can be good for you

We have all heard warnings before about chocolate such as:

"Eating chocolate rots the teeth and makes you fat"

In fact, evidence indicates that, in moderation, chocolate can have health benefits!

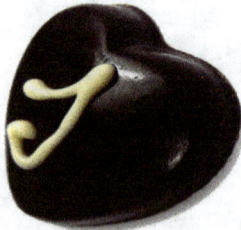

Everybody is aware of the high calorific content of chocolate and the potential for weight gain and obesity. However, in moderation, there are various health benefits attributed to eating chocolate including:

1.   Reduced heart attacks (fewer cardiovascular problems)

2.   Reduced cholesterol levels

3.   Reduced risk of diabetes

4.   Anticancer effects

5.   Reduction of ageing process

6.   Improved neurological/psychological effects

Reduced cholesterol and cardiovascular disease

Many articles describe the beneficial effects of eating chocolate in reducing cardiovascular disease. Most of these, however, are either sensationalised in the popular press to sell newspapers, or they are scientifically flawed, or else the research has been paid for by chocolate manufacturers. However, recently a review published by Dr. Buitrago-Lopez and colleagues (1) has identified seven studies acceptable in terms of meeting high enough scientific standards. From the seven papers, evidence indicated that high chocolate consumption resulted in a 37% reduction in the risk of cardiovascular disease and a 29% reduced risk in the case of strokes.

These favourable effects of chocolate may result from the high content of powerful antioxidants, called flavanoids, in cocoa which give dark chocolate its bitter taste. One such flavanoids, called flavanol, is also present in high concentrations in some fruits and vegetables such as beans, berries and apricots as well as black and green teas and red wine. How flavanols protect the cardiovascular system is debateable but may involve increases in levels of a cell messenger, namely, a gas called nitric oxide.

Nitric oxide is known to improve blood capillary function, lower blood pressure, reduce blood clotting and harmful (LDL)-cholesterol, and increase beneficial (HDL)-cholesterol levels in the blood. All these effects would certainly help prevent the build up of blood clots and furring up of blood vessels leading to cardiovascular disease and strokes. These benefits of chocolate are mainly associated with eating dark chocolate as this has a higher flavanol content than milk chocolate while white chocolate contains no flavanol at all.

Reduced risk of diabetes

Chocolate may also have beneficial effects on diabetes. Type 2 diabetes is characterised by insulin resistance of the cells of the body and increased blood sugar (glucose) levels. Insulin controls uptake of glucose from the blood into the cells for energy production so that when this is disrupted glucose levels rise in the blood. Type 2 diabetes results in increases in levels of harmful cholesterol (LDL), as well as blood clots, heart disease, high blood pressure and kidney damage. Obesity often results in the development of insulin resistance and type 2 diabetes.

Flavanol-rich dark chocolate, but not white chocolate, can reduce insulin resistance in patients. Grassi and colleagues (2) showed that dark chocolate reduces blood pressure and harmful (LDL) cholesterol, as well as improving blood flow and decreasing insulin sensitivity in patients with high blood pressure. Another chemical in cocoa, related to flavanol and called anthocyanin, and present in fruit such as blueberries and acai, has also been shown, in a study of over 200,000 people, to lower the risk of type 2 diabetes (3).

Anticancer effects

Preliminary animal work shows that chocolate may also protect against cancer. In rats fed on a carcinogen (chemical causing cancer) plus cocoa diet, fewer pre-cancerous changes were detectable in the colon than in rats fed on the carcinogen alone. The cocoa-fed animals had improved antioxidant defences as well as less oxidative damage. The latter damage may be a preliminary to development of cancer (4).

Reduction of ageing process - READERS BEWARE!!!!

A typical over-hyped headline appeared recently online entitled "Great news for chocoholics! How eating modified treat can slow down the ageing process" (5). It was announced that the antioxidant flavanols in cocoa had been engineered to be more readily absorbed by the body so that potentially skin oxygenation could be improved to slow the ageing process. The manufacturers, Lycotec Ltd, also describe in their website the modified chocolate not only as "anti-ageing" but also as a "Beauty Chocolate - to enhance skin "glow" and control cellulite inflammation", as well as "Elite Chocolate - to improve muscle oxygenation and performance in sport" (6). The so-called "clinical evidence" was confined to just over 2 lines with no reference to any relevant published scientific article providing proof of the claims. Flavanols may normally be difficult to breakdown and absorb in the gut. The Lycotec technology describes the enhanced uptake into the blood of flavanol from the modified chocolate but no evidence of the anti-ageing claims. Before going out and buying this modified chocolate, which will be available before too long (and probably expensive), wait until the "clinical evidence" is published and reviewed by independent scientists.

Improved neurological/psychological effects

Many other effects have also been ascribed to eating chocolate. These include headaches, mood-swings, sexual arousal, calming, addiction and craving. It is not surprising that some side-effects should be reported since cocoa contains several hundred different chemicals. These chemicals include mimics of cannabis; phenylethylamine which may activate pleasure centres in the brain; caffeine-like stimulants; tryptophan which causes the release of the antidepressant serotonin; as well as endorphins which lessen pain and give feelings of well-being.

Proof for the neurological and psychological effects of chocolate is scarce. One study on the effects of chocolate and cocoa failed to find any such changes following a 6 week diet including 37g dark chocolate per day (7). However, another study (involving a Mars laboratory) has shown that the consumption of cocoa flavanols improves cognitive (mental) processes, maybe due to an increased blood flow (8). Similarly, the intake of flavanoids in chocolate, wine and tea, improved mental processes in 70-74 yr old people in Norway, with wine showing the greatest effect (9).

Many aspects of the possible side effects of chocolate have yet to be examined. Try telling some addicted people that eating chocolate is not a craving and that once eaten there is no feeling of calm, pleasure or euphoria! Maybe the pleasure arises from the smell of chocolate and from the cocoa butter in chocolate which melts in the mouth at about body temperature to form a delicious warm pool of chocolate which then flows down into the stomach to rapidly provide an energy boost from the high fat and sugar content (10).

Risks of eating chocolate

An over-indulgence in chocolate results in weight gain, obesity and associated diseases, as it high in saturated fat and sugar. For example:

50 g of Cadbury's Dairy Milk Chocolate has:

265 Calories, 14.9 g Fat, 9.2 g Saturated Fat, and 28.35 g Sugar

50 g of Tesco Plain Chocolate has:

259 Calories, 13.5 g Fat, 8.5 g Saturated Fat, and 29.2 g Sugar

In other words, a bar of chocolate is composed of over 50% sugar and nearly 30% fat!!!

Exercises to use up the calories in 50g of these chocolates would take about:

Walking 42 min, Swimming 29 min, Cycling 22 min and Running 18 min! (11)

Thus, an over-indulgence in chocolate contributes not only to obesity but also to headaches, cardiovascular problems, diabetes, breast cysts and depression. It is not usually the cocoa causing the problem but the sugar and fat added in making the chocolate. Any food containing such high levels of refined sugar and fat and eaten in large quantities would produce similar health risks. In addition, many of the scientific articles, mentioned above, describing the benefits of chocolate, fed 50 or 100g of chocolate per day to their test subjects. As shown above, a 100g bar of chocolate would contain over 500 extra Calories per day which would be enough to put on 1 pound of fat per week! In order to enjoy the health benefits of eating chocolate, your diet should be rebalanced to take account of the additional Calories. The alternative would be to exercise longer or more vigorously each day, as indicated above. The engineered chocolate being developed by Lycotec Ltd may well mean that the beneficial effects of chocolate can be enjoyed by eating smaller quantities. At present, 10-15 g per day (2-3 squares) of 60% or more cocoa dark chocolate is a reasonable limit to obtain some benefits while avoiding excess Calories.

Reference sources

1.   Buitrago-Lopez   and   colleagues,   BMJ 2011;343:d4488 doi: 10.1136/bmj.d4488.

2. Grassi and colleagues, Hypertension, Vol. 46, pages 398-405, 2005.

3. Wedick and colleagues, American Journal Clinical Nutrition, Vol. 95, pages 925-933, 2012.

4. Rodriguez-Ramiro and colleagues , Molecular Nutrition & Food Research, Vol. 55, pages 1895-1899, 2011.

5. http://dailymail.co.uk/health/article-2150986

6. www.lycotec.com/coco-lycosome.html

7. Crews and colleagues, American Society for Clinical Nutrition, Vol. 87, pages 872-880, 2008.

8. Scholey and colleagues, Journal of Psychopharmacology, Vol. 24, pages 1505-1514, 2010.

9. Nurk and colleagues, The American Institute of Nutrition, Vol. 139, pages 120-127, 2009.

10.www.sciencedaily.com/releases/2008/06/080605150908.html

11. Ratcliffe, "It's Your Life, End the Confusion from Inconsistent Health Advice", Cranmore Publications, 2011.

Chapter 3

Alcohol can be good for you

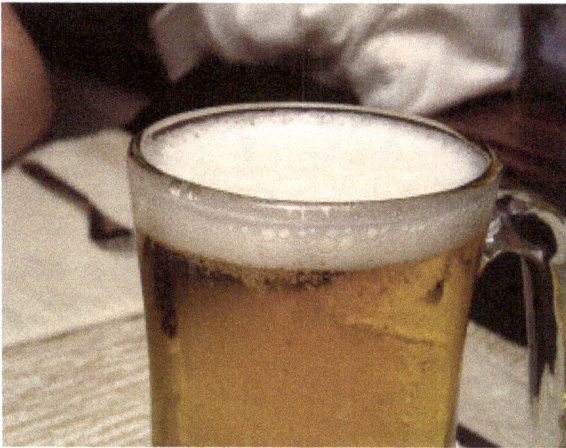

But only if taken in moderation since alcohol is addictive, causes bad behaviour, destroys the liver and breaks up marriages.

Numerous articles have been written about alcohol and, in particular, about the evils of drink. Most people are aware of the health and social problems associated with excessive drinking with many city centres turning into "no-go" areas on Friday and Saturday nights and hospital emergency departments filled with aggressive drunks. However, there is another aspect of alcohol which needs consideration in order to obtain a balanced view and that is the benefits provided from drinking in moderation. These include:

1. Longer life-span

2. Reduced heart attacks (fewer cardiovascular problems)

3. Reduced risk of diabetes

4. Reduced Alzheimer's risk and increased mental (cognitive) ability

5. Miscellaneous benefits

Longer life-span and reduced heart attacks

There is consistent evidence now that people who are either light or moderate drinkers (1-2 drinks per day) have a reduced risk of dying in comparison with non-drinkers and heavy drinkers (3-6 or more daily) (eg. 1). In some of these studies, death rate differences recorded between the groups were very significant. Thus, in the Klatsky paper (1):

The moderate drinkers had half the mortality rate of the heavy drinkers and also had significantly lower death rates than the non-drinkers.

Care, however, must be shown in interpretation of such studies since heavy drinkers are also probably the heaviest smokers with smoking probably contributing to death rates recorded for this group.

Drinking limits

There is concern about setting daily limits for alcohol consumption as it implies that drinking is completely safe whereas the risk of cancer and liver damage increase even in those who drink below recommended limits (eg. 2). At the same time, pregnant women should not drink at all and binge drinkers should allow 48 hr without alcohol for the body to recover. The usual drink limits for men and women are*:

Men Daily Safe Limits: 3-4 units per day

Women Daily Safe Limits: 2-3 units per day

Men Weekly Safe Limits: 21 units per week

Women Weekly Safe Limits: 14 units per week

* There should also be at least two alcohol-free days a week and the weekly units should not be drunk in 1-2 binges per week (3).

Content in *units of various common alcoholic drinks:

Pint or can of normal (Harp) or strong strength (Stella) lager = 2-3 units

Bottle of lager (Budweiser) = 2 units

Pint of ordinary strength (John Smiths) or best (Young's) bitter = 2-3 units

Pint of ordinary (Woodpecker) or strong (Strong-bow) cider = 2-3 units

1 bottle of alcopop (Bacardi Breezer, WKD, Smirnoff Ice) = 2 units

750 ml bottle of wine (check label for strength) = 7-10 units

Large glass wine (250 ml) = 3 units

Standard glass wine (175 ml) = 2 units

Small glass wine (125 ml) = 1.5 units

Small glass champagne (120 ml) = 1.5 units

Single shot of spirit (25 ml), ABV 40% = 1 unit

Tequila shots small or large = 1-1.3 units

Sherry and port (standard pub measure, 50ml) = 1 unit

*These will vary with strength of beer, cider, wine or spirit

The increased longevity of moderate drinkers probably results from the reduction in risk of developing cardiovascular disease, type 2 diabetes, Alzheimer's disease and cognitive decline, as well as other conditions such as arthritis, gallstones, stress and depression (4). For cardiovascular disease and strokes, a recent overview of 84 papers (5) showed that:

• The lowest risk of coronary heart disease occurs in light to moderate drinkers (1-2 drinks per day) who have a reduced risk of about 25% compared with non-drinkers.

• The lowest incidence for strokes is in people with ≤1 (one or less) drinks per day with a reduced risk of 62% compared with the heaviest drinkers of 4 or more drinks per day.

• In addition, moderate alcohol consumption was associated with changes in several healthy blood factors which counteract coronary heart disease, including higher levels of beneficial cholesterol (HDL) (which reduces plaque formation in blood vessels) and adiponectin (a hormone which breaks down fat in the blood and arteries as well as regulating glucose levels), and a reduction in fibrinogen which is involved in blood clotting (6).

• Protection against cardiovascular disease by drinking moderately seems to be most effective in men over 40 yr old and women who have passed the menopause.

Wine, beer or spirits?

Whether wine, beer and spirits have the same protective effect is debateable since wine has consistently been found to reduce cardiovascular risk while beer and spirits are variable in protection reported. However, all alcoholic drinks may provide some degree of protection as it may be the alcohol itself which is protective. Apart from the alcohol, no doubt, the flavanols and anthocyanins and other antioxidants present in wine, dark beer and some whiskeys are, as in chocolate, partially responsible for their protection. Red wine seems to have higher levels of flavanols than white wine but the latter is also protective against cardiovascular disease. The antioxidants in white wine, however, are smaller in size than those in red wine and therefore more easily absorbed by the gut (7).

Reduced risk of diabetes

There is also considerable evidence that, as with cardiovascular disease, moderate drinkers (3-4 per day) are less likely to develop type 2 diabetes than non-drinkers or heavy drinkers (6-8 per day) (eg. 8). Moderate drinking seems to give a 30% or more reduction in the risk of developing type 2 diabetes. The mechanism for this protective effect is not fully understood but may involve the increased insulin sensitivity of subjects drinking moderately (8), so that the control of blood sugar levels would be improved. In heavier drinkers, however, there is evidence of damage to the pancreatic beta cells, which secrete insulin, so that control of blood sugar levels would be lost.

Reduced Alzheimer's risk and increased mental (cognitive) ability

An extensive overview of 143 scientific papers, found that light to moderate drinking in people over 55 yr old results in a 20-25% reduction in the risk of dementia, cognitive decline and impairment. In contrast, in 18-50yr olds there is no such reduction and also no difference in cognition between drinkers and non-drinkers (9). The benefit applied to all forms of dementia including Alzheimer's disease. The protective effect may be better with wine than with beer or spirits but this needs confirmation. The beneficial effects of light to moderate drinking occur in both men and women although men drink more than women and prefer beer and spirits rather than the wine favoured by women.

These results are surprising since drinking any amount of alcohol is generally associated with impaired brain function and mental processes.

The important point is that only light or moderate drinking of no more than 1-3 units per day by people older than 55 produces this protective effect.

Also, the pattern of drinking is important since any protection is lost by binge drinking rather than by a regular light to moderate alcohol intake (10). How light or moderate drinking reduces dementia and mental decline is unknown but may be due to increased beneficial cholesterol (HDL) by alcohol and the reduced risk of blood clots and strokes caused by harmful cholesterol (LDL). Reports exist of a link between cholesterol and the risk of developing dementia but the relationship is complex (11).

Miscellaneous benefits

Apart from the social benefits of light or moderate alcohol consumption, there are other interesting health benefits attributed to drinking alcohol.

These include reductions in the risk and severity of rheumatoid arthritis (12). Di Giuseppe and colleagues (12) showed that women who drank more than 3 glasses of alcohol (60g ethanol) per week over 10 years halved the risk of rheumatoid arthritis, regardless of whether they drank wine, beer or liquor. In addition, drinking weekly about 3-4 units of alcohol can be protective against benign prostate hyperplasia (non-cancerous enlargement of the prostate gland) (13). Much additional work, however, is required on the mechanisms involved in these and the other benefits of drinking alcohol, detailed above.

Risks of drinking alcohol

In conclusion, there are health benefits of drinking light to moderate amounts of alcohol in terms of increased longevity due to reduced risks of heart disease, strokes, type 2 diabetes and dementia. However, alcohol drinking is often abused with 26% men and 18% of women in England exceeding the recommended average weekly limits of 21 and 14 units of alcohol (14). In addition, it is not just the amount of alcohol drunk weekly but the manner of drinking which is important. It is extremely harmful to drink the weekly alcohol limit just in 1-2 binges on a Friday and Saturday night, as so many youngsters seem to do. Alcohol is also addictive with 4% of the population in England aged 16-65 being alcohol-dependent (15) and planning their lives around the next drink. Alcohol addiction is now most common in women of 16-24 yr and men of 25-34 yr old (16).

The bottom line is that a glass or two of alcohol a day may be beneficial, but this can too easily increase and become habit-forming and lead to major health hazards. These hazards can include liver damage, heart problems, strokes, cancer, as well as many social problems. In European men, alcohol consumption results in 10% of all cancers, including cancers of the liver, gut and respiratory tract and, although 1-2 drinks may be beneficial for reducing the risks heart disease, there appears to be no safe lower limit below which alcohol does not induce cancer (17).

Reference sources

1. Klatsky and colleagues, Annals Internal Medicine, Vol. 95, pages 139-145, 1981.

2. Schutze and colleagues, British Medical Journal, BMJ 2011;342:d1584.

3.www.nhs.uk/Livewell/alcohol/Pages/Effectsofalcohol.aspx

4.Power and colleagues, Clinical Biochemistry, Vol. 32, pages 505-518, 1999.

5. Ronskley and colleagues, British Medical Journal, Vol. 342, page 479, 2011.

6. Boivin and colleagues, British Medical Journal, Vol. 342, page 480, 2011.

7. Troup and colleagues, Letter to the Editor, Free radical scavenging abilities of beverages, International Journal of Food Science and Technology, Vol. 30, pages 535 -537, 1995.

8. Crandall and colleagues, The American Journal of Clinical Nutrition, Vol. 90, pages 595-601.

9. Neafsey and Collins, Neuropsychiatric Disease and Treatment, Vol. 7, pages 465–484, 2011.

10. Virta and colleagues, Journal of Alzheimer's Disease, Vol. 22, pages 939-948, 2010.

11. Kaarin and colleagues, American Journal of Geriatric Psychiatry, Vol. 16, pages 343-354, 2008.

12. Di Giuseppe and colleagues, British Medical Journal, BMJ 2012;345:e4230, 2012.

13. Parsons and colleagues, Journal of Urology, Vol. 182, pages 1463-1468, 2009.

14. www.nhs.uk/news/2012/.../Pages/uk-alcohol-deaths-predicted.aspx

15. http://www.nice.org.uk/nicemedia/live/13337/53190/53190.pdf

16. NHS Information Centre, Statistics on Alcohol: England 2009

17. Schutze and colleagues, British Medical Journal, www.bmj.com/content/342/bmj.d1584, 2011.

Final comment

In moderation, sex, chocolate and alcohol can be of benefit to your health so have a drink or two, cover your partner in chocolate and make love!!!!

It's Your Life: End the Confusion from Inconsistent Health Advice

If you are interested in finding out more about a healthy lifestyle and how to remain fit and young then you can find details in my comprehensive book on health: *It's Your Life: End the Confusion from Inconsistent Health Advice.* Here is why the book is unique:

- **It is for people of all different ages,** aiming to optimise health and fitness and maximise an active and independent lifestyle throughout life. It is not a part of the recent deluge of health and diet books or videos produced by B-class "celebrities" but has been written by a biomedical scientist of international repute.

- There are **high impact illustrations** emphasising important points in the text. For example, the cover illustrates the present-day frustration and confusion of the average consumer exposed to contradictory health and dietary advice.

- There are clear summaries of **basic facts for adopting a new health plan.** Thus, for the many people with busy lives who may hate reading health books Chapter 1 ("Food, The Basic Diet"), Chapter 9 ("Exercise, Basic Introduction") and other Chapters are designed for rapid reference, often to specific age-groups of people.

- You will also not find in most other books descriptions of how many aspects of **diet and exercise change at different times of life** (Chapter 1) as well as reasons for weight gain as we age and advice as how to avoid this (Chapter 2, "Help! What Am I Eating?").

- There are **extensive tables for rapid identification of foods containing high levels of calories, saturated fats, salt and sugar** (Chapter 2). Thus, information on over 300 different food groups can be extracted at a glance without the necessity of reading minute and confusing Supermarket Food Labels.

- You will also not find in most books **not only clearly tabulated facts** about "**The Good, The Bad And The Ugly Fats**", and "**Fibre**" but also appraisals of the Atkins and GI "**Fad Diets**" (Chapter 3).

- **Details of the rates of pesticide contamination of fruit, vegetables and other types of food** using easily interpreted tables are also given (Chapter 4). A summary table is also included, for attaching to the refrigerator door or notice board, to identify **the least chemically polluted foods.**

- **A list is given of which organic foods are the most important to buy** (Chapter 4) and an explanation why, in these financially challenged times, it is **unnecessary** to eat just organic foods.

- Details are also given **of the potential impact on food safety of Food Additives, Preservatives and Colourants** (Chapter 5) together with consideration of the **total chemical loading** of the body from all sources (Chapter 6, "The Cocktail Effect"). Possible interactions of chemicals accumulated from pesticides and additives in food, and from cosmetics and household sources, are also discussed, and advice is given on **reducing the uptake of chemicals from the environment**.

- You will also not find in other books an understanding of the **"Vitamin Dilemma" as "To Take Or Not To Take, That Is The Question"** (Chapters 7 and 8) facing most people following conflicting advice in the media. Clear scientific analysis of the latest research shows that people require different supplements at different stages in their lives. **Supplement recommendations are made for each stage from pregnancy to old age.**

- There is also **an understanding of the "To Gym Or Not To Gym-That Is The Question" dilemma faced by many people beginning to exercise for the first time** (Chapter 9). It introduces the basics and benefits of regular exercise, describes how to begin training in the gym, and provides an outline exercise programme (Chapter 10).

- **Details of "Alternative Types Of Exercise For Gym–Haters"** (Chapter 11), with different sports and activities are also described together with the calories used and **a table of the time taken with different sports to burn off highly calorific snacks.** Uniquely, the effects of each type of exercise are presented in terms of joint damage and cardiovascular function, and **advice on exercising at different ages** is also included.

- In summary, **"IT'S YOUR LIFE"**, presents the best advice available for optimising health and fitness in a manner designed to enlighten and engage the non-expert reader.

You can find details of where to buy the book here:

http://www.cranmorepublications.co.uk/6

In order to receive the latest health advice simply enter your email address here:

http://endtheconfusion.wordpress.com

Other Books by the Author:

IT'S YOUR LIFE – END THE CONFUSION FROM INCONSISTENT HEALTH ADVICE

IT'S YOUR LIFE – A HEALTHY DIET MADE EASY

IT'S YOUR LIFE – AVOIDING HARMFUL CHEMICALS IN YOUR FOOD

IT'S YOUR LIFE – AVOID THE COCKTAIL EFFECT OF HARMFUL CHEMICALS IN YOUR BODY

IT'S YOUR LIFE – VITAMINS & SUPPLEMENTS FOR ALL AGES

IT'S YOUR LIFE – EXERCISE FOR ALL AGES

KEEPING MOTHER, BABY AND CHILD SAFE FROM TOXIC CHEMICALS